GALLBLADDER DIET AFTER REMOVAL

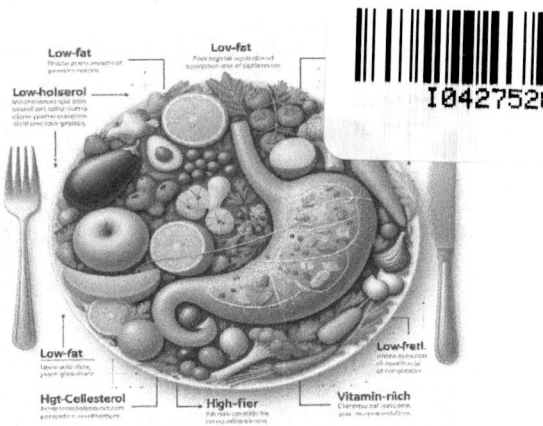

A Collection of Nourishing Recipes and an Approved Grocery List for a Post-Gallbladder Removal Recovery Journey

Tina Feldman

TABLE OF CONTENTS

PART 1

INTRODUCTION

Once upon a time in a quaint little town, there lived a man named John who had recently undergone gallbladder removal surgery. Despite the successful procedure, John found himself facing a new challenge—adjusting to life without his gallbladder.

In the days following the surgery, John's doctor emphasized the significance of adopting a gallbladder-friendly diet. Understanding the importance of this dietary adjustment, John decided to embark on a journey of culinary exploration.

The first few days were a delicate phase for John. He started with a clear liquid diet, gradually introducing broths to nourish his body and aid in the recovery process. John's dedication to following the immediate post-surgery diet guidelines was unwavering, and it played a crucial role in preventing any complications.

As the initial days passed, John continued to adhere to the recommended dietary plan, focusing on easily digestible and low-fat foods. He discovered the pleasure of sipping on herbal teas, indulging in smoothies, and relishing the comfort of well-prepared broths. These choices not only provided him with essential nutrients but also eased the transition into his new post-surgery reality.

With time, John began reintroducing soft foods into his diet. He savored the simplicity of mashed potatoes, steamed vegetables, and poached chicken. These choices were gentle on his digestive system, allowing him to regain his strength without overwhelming his body.

John's commitment to his gallbladder diet didn't stop at the immediate post-surgery phase. Recognizing the long-term adjustments needed, he started incorporating a variety of nutrient-rich foods into his meals. Fruits, vegetables, lean proteins, and whole grains became staples in his diet, supporting his overall health.

As the weeks turned into months, John's dedication bore fruit. He felt energized, his digestive discomfort diminished, and he discovered a renewed sense of well-being. The lifestyle adjustments he made weren't just about following dietary guidelines but about embracing a holistic approach to health.

John's story became an inspiration for others facing similar challenges. His journey highlighted the importance of personalized, post-gallbladder removal dietary adjustments and demonstrated that with mindful choices, one could navigate this new chapter with resilience and optimism.

Understanding the Gallbladder and Its Role

The gallbladder is a small, pear-shaped organ located beneath the liver in the upper right part of the abdomen. Despite its relatively modest size, the gallbladder plays a crucial role in the digestive system. Understanding its anatomy and functions is essential for appreciating its importance in overall health.

Anatomy of the Gallbladder:
Location:
- The gallbladder is positioned below the liver on the right side of the abdomen.
- It is connected to the liver and the small intestine through a series of ducts, including the common bile duct.

Structure:
- The gallbladder is typically about 3-4 inches long and holds approximately 50 milliliters of bile.
- It has a neck, body, and fundus, and its inner surface is lined with a mucous membrane.
- Role of the Gallbladder:

Bile Storage:
- The primary function of the gallbladder is to store bile, a digestive fluid produced by the liver.
- Bile is essential for the digestion and absorption of fats.

Bile Release:
- When food, especially fatty food, enters the small intestine, the gallbladder contracts and releases bile into the common bile duct.
- Bile then flows into the small intestine, where it helps emulsify fats, breaking them down into smaller particles for easier digestion by enzymes.

Fat Digestion:
- Bile contains bile salts, which aid in the digestion and absorption of fats.
- Bile salts surround fat particles, creating smaller droplets that pancreatic lipase enzymes can break down more efficiently.

Nutrient Absorption:
- The breakdown of fats in the presence of bile allows the absorption of fat-soluble vitamins (A, D, E, and K) and other essential nutrients.

Common Gallbladder Issues:

Gallstones:
- Gallstones are solid particles that form in the gallbladder due to an imbalance in the substances that make up bile.
- These stones can cause pain, inflammation, and blockages in the gallbladder or bile ducts.

Cholecystitis:
- Inflammation of the gallbladder, often caused by gallstones, can lead to a condition called cholecystitis.
- Symptoms include abdominal pain, nausea, and vomiting.

Gallbladder Removal (Cholecystectomy):
- In cases of severe gallbladder issues, a common medical intervention is the removal of the gallbladder.
- Despite its removal, most individuals can continue to digest fats adequately due to the continuous secretion of bile from the liver into the small intestine.

Lifestyle Impact:
Dietary Considerations:
- Individuals without a gallbladder may experience changes in fat digestion.
- It is often recommended to consume smaller, well-distributed meals throughout the day and to avoid excessive fat intake in a single meal.

Adaptation:
The body can adapt to the absence of the gallbladder, and individuals can lead normal, healthy lives with proper dietary adjustments.
Understanding the role of the gallbladder helps individuals appreciate the importance of maintaining digestive health and making informed choices in diet and lifestyle. For specific concerns or conditions

related to the gallbladder, consulting with a healthcare professional is crucial for personalized advice and treatment options

Immediate Post-Surgery Diet Guidelines (First Few Days)

Clear liquids and broths

Following surgery, it is essential to adhere to a carefully planned diet to facilitate the healing process and avoid any complications. The immediate post-surgery period, typically the first few days, often requires patients to follow a clear liquid and broth diet as part of their recovery plan.

Clear liquids and broths serve several purposes during this crucial stage of recovery:

Hydration: Clear liquids, such as water, clear juices, and broth, help maintain hydration levels, which is vital for the body's overall function. Staying hydrated aids in preventing complications such as constipation and supports the healing process.

Easy to Digest: After surgery, the digestive system may be sensitive and less active. Clear liquids and broths are easy on the digestive system, reducing the risk of nausea, vomiting, or discomfort. This allows the body to absorb essential nutrients without placing undue stress on the gastrointestinal tract.

Electrolyte Balance: Broths, especially if they contain sodium and potassium, can help restore electrolyte balance, which may be disrupted during surgery. Electrolytes are crucial for maintaining proper fluid balance, nerve function, and muscle contractions.

Provides Necessary Nutrients: While clear liquids and broths are not as nutrient-dense as solid foods, they still provide some essential nutrients. Broths, for example, may offer proteins, vitamins, and minerals, albeit in a more easily digestible form.

Minimizes Surgical Stress: Post-surgery, the body is in a state of stress, and consuming easily digestible liquids reduces the energy expenditure required for digestion. This allows the body to redirect energy towards the healing process and overall recovery.

It's important to note that individual dietary recommendations may vary based on the type of surgery and the patient's overall health. Always follow the specific guidelines provided by the surgical team or healthcare professional.

Typically, the immediate post-surgery diet may include:

- Clear Liquids: Water, clear broths, herbal teas, clear fruit juices (without pulp), and sports drinks without added colors.

- Broths: Chicken, beef, or vegetable broths are commonly recommended. These can be enriched with extra nutrients and electrolytes for added benefits.

It is crucial to progress from clear liquids to more substantial foods gradually. As the patient's tolerance and appetite improve, healthcare providers may advance the diet to include full liquids, soft foods, and eventually a regular diet

Gradually reintroducing soft foods

The gradual reintroduction of soft foods in the immediate post-surgery period is a critical step in transitioning from a clear liquid and broth diet to a more diverse and nutrient-dense eating plan. This phase typically occurs a few days after surgery and is carefully monitored by healthcare professionals to ensure the patient's comfort and minimize the risk of complications. Here are details about reintroducing soft foods during the first few days of the post-surgery diet:

Timing and Progression:
- The timing for advancing to soft foods depends on the individual's recovery and the type of surgery performed.
- Generally, healthcare providers will assess the patient's tolerance to clear liquids, monitor signs of gastrointestinal function, and then gradually introduce soft foods as appropriate.

Soft Food Options:

- Mashed Vegetables: Potatoes, sweet potatoes, carrots, and other root vegetables can be boiled and mashed to create a soft texture.
- Applesauce: Unsweetened applesauce is easy to digest and provides some natural sweetness.
- Yogurt: Plain, low-fat yogurt without added sugars can be a good source of protein and probiotics.
- Pudding: Smooth and creamy puddings without chunks can be a tasty option.
- Cottage Cheese: Soft and easily digestible, cottage cheese is a good source of protein.
- Oatmeal: Cooked oatmeal provides fiber and can be easily modified for texture.
- Scrambled Eggs: Soft, scrambled eggs are a good source of protein.
- Soups with Soft Ingredients: Gradually transitioning from clear broths to soups with soft vegetables or noodles can be beneficial.

Texture Modifications:

- Foods should be well-cooked and soft in texture to avoid any strain on the digestive system.
- Gravy, sauces, or broth can be added to enhance moisture and flavor.
- Chewing should be minimized during this phase to prevent any discomfort.

Portion Control:
- Start with small, frequent meals to gauge the body's response.
- Monitor for any signs of nausea, vomiting, or discomfort after introducing new soft foods.

Hydration:
- Continue to prioritize hydration during the soft food phase.
- Adequate fluid intake aids in digestion and helps prevent complications such as constipation.
- Nutrient Considerations:
- Soft foods should still focus on providing essential nutrients, including protein, vitamins, and minerals, to support the healing process.

Individualized Approach:

- The reintroduction of soft foods is highly individualized, taking into account the patient's medical history, dietary preferences, and the specific surgical procedure.
- Patients should follow the guidance of their healthcare team closely and communicate any concerns or adverse reactions. The goal is to gradually restore normal eating patterns while promoting healing and minimizing any post-surgery complications. As the patient progresses and demonstrates tolerance for soft foods, the diet can be further advanced to

include a broader range of textures and food types.

Importance of hydration

Hydration is of paramount importance in the immediate post-surgery period, particularly during the first few days, as it plays a crucial role in the overall recovery and well-being of the patient. Adequate hydration is essential for various physiological functions, and its significance is heightened during the initial stages of the post-surgery diet. Here's why maintaining proper hydration is vital in the immediate post-surgery period:

Supports Healing Process:

Hydration is essential for tissue repair and the healing of surgical incisions. An adequately hydrated body ensures optimal circulation, allowing nutrients and oxygen to reach the surgical site efficiently.

Prevents Complications:

Dehydration can increase the risk of post-surgery complications such as constipation, urinary tract infections, and electrolyte imbalances. These complications may hinder the recovery process and lead to additional discomfort for the patient.

Optimizes Medication Absorption:

Many post-surgery patients are prescribed medications to manage pain, prevent infection, and aid in recovery. Proper hydration supports the absorption and effectiveness of these medications.

Reduces Nausea and Dizziness:
Dehydration can contribute to feelings of nausea and dizziness, which may already be present as side effects of anesthesia or the surgical procedure. Maintaining adequate fluid intake can help alleviate these symptoms.

Enhances Gastrointestinal Function:
Hydration supports healthy gastrointestinal function, preventing constipation and promoting the smooth passage of food through the digestive system. This is particularly important as the diet progresses from clear liquids to soft foods.

Regulates Body Temperature:
Surgical procedures, anesthesia, and the healing process can impact the body's temperature regulation. Staying well-hydrated assists in maintaining a stable body temperature, preventing overheating or hypothermia.

Minimizes Kidney Strain:
Adequate hydration is crucial for maintaining kidney function, especially when patients are receiving medications or undergoing procedures that may place additional strain on the kidneys.

Boosts Energy Levels:
Recovery from surgery can be physically demanding, and staying hydrated ensures an adequate supply of energy to the body. This is

essential for the patient to regain strength and mobility.

Facilitates Nutrient Transport:
Hydration is necessary for the transport of essential nutrients throughout the body. This is critical for providing the necessary building blocks for cellular repair and regeneration.

Improves Overall Comfort:
- Proper hydration contributes to overall comfort and well-being. It helps alleviate common post-surgery symptoms such as dry mouth and throat, making the recovery experience more manageable for the patient.
- Patients are usually encouraged to start with clear liquids and progress to more substantial fluids as tolerated. Healthcare providers closely monitor fluid intake and may adjust recommendations based on the individual patient's needs. It is essential for patients to follow the hydration guidelines provided by their medical team to support a smooth and successful recovery after surgery.

Foods to avoid initially

In the immediate post-surgery period, it's crucial to follow dietary guidelines that prioritize the healing process and minimize the risk of complications. Certain foods can be more challenging for the body to tolerate during the first few days after surgery, and it's advisable to avoid or limit the intake of the following:

Solid Foods:
Initially, solid foods should be avoided, as the digestive system may be sensitive and less active immediately after surgery. The focus is on gradually reintroducing softer textures.

Spicy and Highly Seasoned Foods:
Spicy and heavily seasoned foods may irritate the digestive tract. It's best to avoid these during the initial post-surgery days to minimize any potential discomfort.

Hard or Crunchy Foods:
Foods that are hard or crunchy, such as raw vegetables, nuts, and seeds, can be challenging to digest and may pose a risk of irritation or blockage, especially if the surgery involves the digestive system.

Fibrous Foods:
High-fiber foods like whole grains, beans, and certain fruits and vegetables should be avoided initially. These can be harder to digest and may contribute to gas and bloating.

Dairy Products:
Some people may experience lactose intolerance or difficulty digesting dairy products immediately after surgery. It's advisable to limit or avoid dairy until tolerance is assessed.

Carbonated Beverages:
Carbonated drinks can cause gas and bloating. Opting for non-carbonated and non-caffeinated beverages is recommended to avoid any additional discomfort.

Alcohol:
Alcohol can interfere with medications, dehydrate the body, and potentially interact with the healing process. It's advisable to avoid alcohol during the initial recovery period.

Highly Sugary Foods:
Foods and beverages with high sugar content may not provide the necessary nutrients for recovery and can contribute to fluctuations in blood sugar levels.

Caffeine:
Caffeine can have diuretic effects, potentially leading to dehydration. It's recommended to limit or avoid caffeinated beverages during the early post-surgery phase.

Processed or Fried Foods:
Processed and fried foods may be harder to digest and can contribute to inflammation. Opting for simple, whole foods is generally recommended.

Red Meat:
Red meat can be harder to digest than lighter protein sources. Initially focusing on lean protein sources like poultry or fish is often advised.

Seeds and Nuts:
Small seeds and nuts may be difficult to digest and can pose a choking hazard. It's advisable to avoid them until the digestive system has had time to recover.

Long-term success in managing a post-gallbladder removal diet

lifestyle modifications

Long-term dietary adjustments are often necessary for individuals who have undergone gallbladder removal surgery, a procedure known as cholecystectomy. The gallbladder plays a role in bile storage and concentration, aiding in the digestion of fats. After its removal, some people may experience changes in digestion and dietary tolerance. Making lifestyle adjustments to accommodate these changes can help maintain digestive comfort and overall well-being. Here are some long-term dietary adjustments for a post-gallbladder removal diet:

Gradual Introduction of Fats:
After gallbladder surgery, some individuals may experience difficulty digesting fats. Gradually reintroduce healthy fats into the diet, such as avocados, olive oil, and fatty fish, to allow the digestive system to adjust.

Emphasis on Low-Fat Foods:
Opt for a diet that is lower in saturated and trans fats. Choose lean proteins, such as poultry, fish, and legumes, and incorporate whole grains, fruits, and vegetables into meals.

Frequent, Smaller Meals:
Eating smaller, more frequent meals throughout the day can help manage digestion and reduce the likelihood of overwhelming the digestive system with a large amount of food at once.

Hydration:
Staying well-hydrated is essential for digestion and overall health. Adequate water intake supports the body's ability to process and absorb nutrients efficiently.

Fiber-Rich Foods:
Include fiber-rich foods in the diet to support digestive health. Whole grains, fruits, vegetables, and legumes are good sources of dietary fiber. However, it's essential to introduce fiber gradually to avoid excessive gas and bloating.

Limit Gas-Producing Foods:
Some individuals may experience increased gas after gallbladder removal. Limiting gas-producing foods, such as beans, broccoli, cabbage, and carbonated beverages, may help alleviate this symptom.

Monitoring Dairy Intake:
Some people may experience temporary lactose intolerance after gallbladder removal. Monitor dairy intake and consider lactose-free options if needed.

Avoiding Trigger Foods:
Identify and avoid foods that may trigger digestive discomfort. Common trigger foods include spicy, greasy, and heavily processed items.

Moderating Coffee and Caffeine:
Coffee and caffeine can stimulate bile production. While moderate intake may be well-tolerated, excessive consumption could lead to digestive discomfort.

Individualized Approach:
Every individual's tolerance to different foods varies. Pay attention to personal responses and tailor the diet based on individual needs and preferences.

Supplement Consideration:
Some individuals may benefit from digestive enzyme supplements to aid in the breakdown of fats. Consult with a healthcare professional before incorporating any supplements into the diet.

Regular Monitoring:
Regularly monitor how dietary adjustments affect digestion and overall well-being. Keep a food diary to identify patterns and discuss any concerns with a healthcare provider.

Ongoing communication with healthcare providers

Ongoing communication with healthcare providers is crucial for individuals adapting to long-term dietary adjustments after gallbladder removal surgery. Continuous dialogue ensures that the post-operative dietary plan aligns with the individual's specific needs, promotes optimal health, and addresses any emerging concerns. Here are key aspects of maintaining open communication with healthcare professionals in the context of a post-gallbladder removal diet:

Follow-Up Appointments:
Attend scheduled follow-up appointments with the surgical team or healthcare provider to discuss recovery progress and address any post-operative concerns.
Share details about dietary habits, any digestive issues, and overall well-being during these appointments.

Symptom Monitoring:
Actively monitor and report any digestive symptoms, such as bloating, gas, diarrhea, or discomfort after meals. This information helps healthcare providers tailor dietary recommendations to individual needs.

Nutritional Guidance:
Seek ongoing nutritional guidance from registered dietitians or nutritionists to ensure that dietary adjustments align with long-term health goals.

Discuss any challenges or concerns related to maintaining a balanced and nutritious diet without the gallbladder.

Medication Adjustments:
Inform healthcare providers about any medications taken, especially those related to digestion or nutrient absorption. Medication adjustments may be necessary to support the altered digestive process post-gallbladder removal.

Fluid Intake:
Discuss fluid intake and hydration needs to ensure that the body remains adequately hydrated. Proper hydration is essential for digestion and overall health.

Review of Dietary Progress:
Regularly review dietary progress and discuss any changes in tolerance to specific foods or food groups. This information helps healthcare providers make informed recommendations for long-term dietary adjustments.

Weight Management:
If weight management is a concern, collaborate with healthcare professionals to develop a balanced and sustainable approach to achieving and maintaining a healthy weight without compromising nutrient intake.

Supplement Guidance:
Discuss the use of any supplements, including digestive enzymes, bile acid supplements, or multivitamins. Healthcare providers can provide guidance on appropriate supplementation based on individual needs.

Educational Resources:
Request educational resources or materials to enhance understanding of the digestive process post-gallbladder removal. This knowledge empowers individuals to make informed dietary choices.

Psychosocial Support:
Discuss any psychosocial aspects of dietary adjustments, such as emotional or psychological challenges related to the surgery or changes in eating habits. Healthcare providers can offer additional support or refer individuals to appropriate resources.

Long-Term Health Monitoring:
Ongoing communication allows healthcare providers to monitor long-term health outcomes and make any necessary adjustments to support overall well-being.

Individualized Care Plans:
Collaborate with healthcare providers to create individualized care plans that consider personal preferences, lifestyle factors, and health goals.

Kitchen preparation guide for post gallbladder removal

Adapting your kitchen and cooking habits after gallbladder removal is essential to support a smooth transition to a post-surgery diet. The following details cover key aspects of kitchen preparation for individuals who have undergone gallbladder removal:

Stocking the Pantry:
Prioritize a pantry stocked with easily digestible, low-fat foods. Include items such as:
Whole grains: Rice, quinoa, and oats.
Low-fat proteins: Canned or pouched tuna, salmon, lean meats, and legumes.
Low-residue foods: White bread, crackers, and low-fiber cereals.

Healthy Cooking Oils:
Opt for cooking oils that are easier to digest. Olive oil, canola oil, and coconut oil are good choices. Use these oils in moderation to reduce the risk of overwhelming the digestive system with fats.

Cooking Methods:
Choose gentle cooking methods that minimize the need for added fats. Steaming, baking, grilling, and boiling are preferable to deep frying.
Invest in non-stick cookware to reduce the need for excessive cooking oils.

Herbs and Spices:
Embrace herbs and mild spices to add flavor to meals without relying on heavy sauces or excessive seasoning. Common choices include basil, oregano, thyme, and mild spices like cumin or cinnamon.

Low-Fat Dairy Alternatives:
If dairy tolerance is an issue, explore low-fat or lactose-free dairy alternatives, such as almond or coconut milk, and yogurt made from these alternatives.

Lean Proteins:
Include lean protein sources, such as poultry, fish, eggs, and tofu. These are easier to digest compared to fatty cuts of meat.

Fruits and Vegetables:
Choose easily digestible fruits and vegetables. Consider options like peeled and cooked apples, bananas, carrots, and zucchini. Gradually reintroduce fiber-rich options as tolerated.

Meal Preparation:
Prepare meals in smaller portions to allow for more frequent, manageable eating throughout the day.
Invest in portion control tools, such as measuring cups, to monitor food intake.

Hydration Station:
Keep a water bottle accessible to encourage regular hydration. Proper hydration supports digestion and overall health.

Avoiding Trigger Foods:
Identify and eliminate trigger foods that may cause digestive discomfort. Common triggers include spicy foods, fatty cuts of meat, and processed foods.

Meal Planning:
Plan meals in advance to ensure a balance of nutrients and variety in the diet. This reduces the reliance on convenience or processed foods.

Food Diary:
Maintain a food diary to track dietary choices, symptoms, and overall well-being. This can help identify patterns and make informed adjustments with the guidance of healthcare providers.

Gradual Reintroduction:
Gradually reintroduce foods into the diet to assess tolerance. Begin with clear liquids, progress to soft foods, and then incorporate more diverse textures as recommended by healthcare providers.

Kitchen Organization:
Organize the kitchen to make meal preparation more efficient and enjoyable. Clear clutter and ensure that utensils and cookware are easily accessible.

Consulting a Dietitian:
Consider consulting with a registered dietitian who can provide personalized advice and meal plans tailored to individual dietary needs and preferences.

Essential kitchen and cooking tools for gallbladder removal diet

Adapting to a gallbladder removal diet may require some adjustments in your kitchen. Here's a list of essential kitchen and cooking tools that can make the transition easier:

Non-Stick Cookware:
Non-stick pans and pots reduce the need for excessive cooking oils, making it easier to control fat intake.

Steamer Basket:
A steamer basket is ideal for gently cooking vegetables, making them easier to digest without losing essential nutrients.

Blender or Food Processor:
Useful for creating smooth soups, purees, and sauces that are easier on the digestive system.

Sharp Knives:
Invest in sharp knives to make cutting and preparing fruits, vegetables, and lean proteins more efficient.

Measuring Cups and Spoons:
Portion control is crucial, especially during the initial stages of adjusting to the post-gallbladder removal diet. Measuring tools help manage food intake.

Slow Cooker or Crockpot:
These allow for easy preparation of well-cooked, tender meals without the need for excessive fats.

Vegetable Peeler:
Useful for peeling vegetables and fruits, making them easier to digest.

Lactose-Free or Low-Lactose Dairy Alternatives:
If lactose intolerance is a concern, having alternatives like almond or coconut milk and yogurt on hand can be beneficial.

Hydration Tools:
Water bottles or hydration systems to encourage regular fluid intake, crucial for digestion and overall health.

Food Diary or Meal Planning Apps:
Keep a food diary or use meal planning apps to track dietary choices, symptoms, and overall well-being. This can help identify patterns and make informed adjustments.

Portion Control Plates:
Specialty plates with sections for proteins, vegetables, and carbohydrates can aid in managing portion sizes.

Strainer or Colander:
Useful for draining and rinsing canned goods and cooked foods.

Spatulas and Ladles:
Non-metallic spatulas and ladles for use with non-stick cookware to prevent scratching.

Cutting Boards:
Separate cutting boards for different food groups (meats, vegetables, fruits) to prevent cross-contamination.

Cooking Utensils:
Wooden or silicone cooking utensils that won't scratch non-stick surfaces.

Thermometer:
A food thermometer ensures that meats are cooked thoroughly without overcooking.

Herb and Spice Containers:
Keep a well-stocked supply of herbs and mild spices to add flavor without excessive seasoning.

Meal Storage Containers:
Prepare and store meals in easily reheatable containers for convenience.

Cooking Oils:
Opt for healthy cooking oils like olive oil, canola oil, and coconut oil to manage fat intake.

Nutrient Supplements:
If advised by healthcare professionals, consider keeping any recommended supplements or digestive aids in your kitchen.

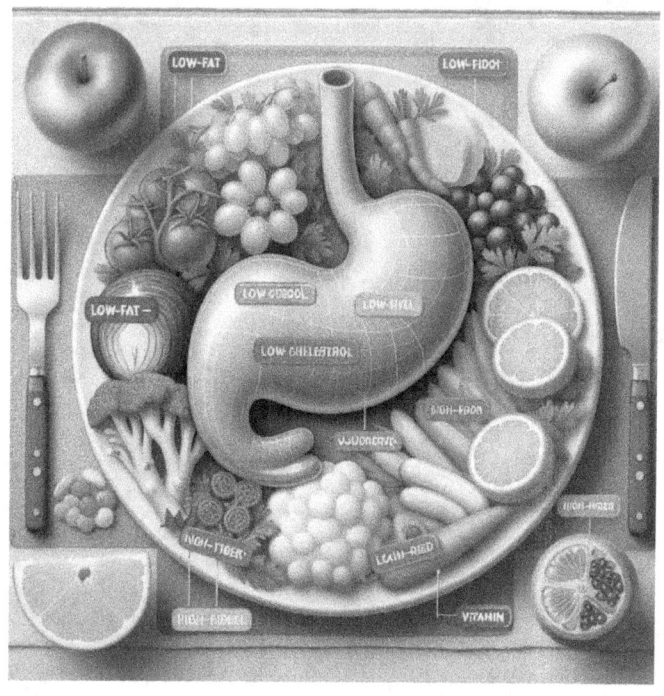

PART 2

ESSENTIAL GALLBLADDER FRIENDLY GROCERY LIST

Fruits

Apples:
Recommended Daily Fat Intake: Less than 30% of daily caloric intake from fat.
Fiber Content: Approximately 4 grams per medium-sized apple.
Calories: Around 95 calories per medium-sized apple.
Serving Size: 1 medium-sized apple.

Berries (Strawberries, Blueberries, Raspberries):
Recommended Daily Fat Intake: Less than 30% of daily caloric intake from fat.
Fiber Content: Varies by berry; approximately 3-4 grams per cup.
Calories: Around 50-80 calories per cup.
Serving Size: 1 cup of berries.

Bananas:
Recommended Daily Fat Intake: Less than 30% of daily caloric intake from fat.
Fiber Content: Approximately 3 grams per medium-sized banana.
Calories: Around 105 calories per medium-sized banana.
Serving Size: 1 medium-sized banana.

Pears:
Recommended Daily Fat Intake: Less than 30% of daily caloric intake from fat.
Fiber Content: Approximately 6 grams per medium-sized pear.
Calories: Around 100 calories per medium-sized pear.
Serving Size: 1 medium-sized pear.

Papaya:
Recommended Daily Fat Intake: Less than 30% of daily caloric intake from fat.
Fiber Content: Approximately 5 grams per cup.
Calories: Around 60 calories per cup.
Serving Size: 1 cup of papaya cubes.

Melons (Cantaloupe, Honeydew):
Recommended Daily Fat Intake: Less than 30% of daily caloric intake from fat.
Fiber Content: Approximately 1-2 grams per cup.
Calories: Around 60-70 calories per cup.
Serving Size: 1 cup of melon cubes.

Peaches:
Recommended Daily Fat Intake: Less than 30% of daily caloric intake from fat.
Fiber Content: Approximately 3 grams per medium-sized peach.
Calories: Around 60 calories per medium-sized peach.
Serving Size: 1 medium-sized peach.

Grapes:
Recommended Daily Fat Intake: Less than 30% of daily caloric intake from fat.
Fiber Content: Approximately 1 gram per cup.
Calories: Around 60-70 calories per cup.
Serving Size: 1 cup of grapes.

Watermelon:
Recommended Daily Fat Intake: Less than 30% of daily caloric intake from fat.
Fiber Content: Approximately 1 gram per cup.
Calories: Around 45 calories per cup.
Serving Size: 1 cup of watermelon cubes.

Kiwi:
Recommended Daily Fat Intake: Less than 30% of daily caloric intake from fat.
Fiber Content: Approximately 2.1 grams per medium-sized kiwi.
Calories: Around 50 calories per medium-sized kiwi.
Serving Size: 1 medium-sized kiwi

Vegetable

Spinach:
Serving Size: 1 cup raw
Calories: Approximately 7 calories
Fiber: About 1 gram
Fat: Minimal
Notes: Spinach is a low-calorie, nutrient-dense leafy green.

Zucchini:
Serving Size: 1 cup sliced
Calories: Approximately 20 calories
Fiber: Around 2 grams
Fat: Very low
Notes: Zucchini is low in calories and easy to digest.

Carrots:
Serving Size: 1 medium carrot
Calories: Approximately 25 calories
Fiber: About 2 grams
Fat: Minimal
Notes: Carrots are a good source of beta-carotene and low in fat.

Bell Peppers:
Serving Size: 1 medium pepper
Calories: Approximately 25 calories
Fiber: About 3 grams
Fat: Very low
Notes: Bell peppers are rich in vitamins and low in fat.

Cucumbers:
Serving Size: 1 cup sliced
Calories: Approximately 15 calories
Fiber: About 1 gram
Fat: Minimal
Notes: Cucumbers are hydrating and low in both calories and fat.

Broccoli:
Serving Size: 1 cup chopped
Calories: Approximately 30 calories
Fiber: Around 2.5 grams
Fat: Minimal
Notes: Broccoli is a nutrient-dense vegetable with moderate fiber content.

Cauliflower:
Serving Size: 1 cup chopped
Calories: Approximately 25 calories
Fiber: About 2 grams
Fat: Very low
Notes: Cauliflower is versatile and low in both calories and fat.

Leafy Greens (Kale, Swiss Chard):
Serving Size: 1 cup raw
Calories: Approximately 7-10 calories (varies)
Fiber: About 1-2 grams (varies)
Fat: Minimal
Notes: Leafy greens are nutrient-rich and low in both calories and fat.

Sweet Potatoes:
Serving Size: 1 medium sweet potato
Calories: Approximately 100 calories
Fiber: Around 4 grams
Fat: Minimal
Notes: Sweet potatoes are a good source of fiber and vitamins.

Asparagus:
Serving Size: 1 cup cooked
Calories: Approximately 40 calories
Fiber: About 4 grams
Fat: Very low
Notes: Asparagus is low in calories and a good source of fiber.

Lean protein

Chicken Breast:
Serving Size: 3 ounces cooked
Calories: Approximately 165 calories
Protein: About 31 grams
Fat: 3.6 grams
Notes: Skinless, boneless chicken breast is a lean protein option.

Turkey (Lean Ground):
Serving Size: 3 ounces cooked
Calories: Approximately 135 calories
Protein: About 20 grams
Fat: 7 grams
Notes: Choose lean ground turkey for lower fat content.

Fish (Salmon, Trout, Cod):
Serving Size: 3 ounces cooked
Calories: Varies (e.g., salmon: 155 calories)
Protein: About 20-25 grams
Fat: Varies (e.g., salmon: 8 grams)
Notes: Fatty fish like salmon provide healthy omega-3 fatty acids.

Lean Beef (Sirloin, Tenderloin):
Serving Size: 3 ounces cooked
Calories: Approximately 150 calories
Protein: About 26 grams
Fat: 6 grams
Notes: Choose lean cuts of beef to minimize fat intake.

Pork (Tenderloin):
Serving Size: 3 ounces cooked
Calories: Approximately 120 calories
Protein: About 22 grams
Fat: 3 grams
Notes: Pork tenderloin is a lean cut with lower fat content.

Eggs:
Serving Size: 2 large eggs
Calories: Approximately 140 calories
Protein: About 12 grams
Fat: 10 grams
Notes: Eggs are a versatile protein source with healthy fats.

Tofu:
Serving Size: 1/2 cup (cubed)
Calories: Approximately 94 calories
Protein: About 10 grams
Fat: 6 grams
Notes: Tofu is a plant-based protein option with moderate fat content.

Cottage Cheese (Low-Fat):
Serving Size: 1/2 cup
Calories: Approximately 80 calories
Protein: About 14 grams
Fat: 1 gram
Notes: Low-fat cottage cheese is a good source of protein with minimal fat.

Greek Yogurt (Low-Fat):
Serving Size: 1 cup
Calories: Approximately 100 calories
Protein: About 15 grams
Fat: 2 grams
Notes: Choose low-fat Greek yogurt for a protein-rich dairy option.

Lentils:
Serving Size: 1 cup cooked
Calories: Approximately 230 calories
Protein: About 18 grams
Fat: 1 gram
Notes: Lentils are a plant-based protein with high fiber content.

Healthy fats

Avocado:
Serving Size: 1/2 medium avocado
Calories: Approximately 120 calories
Healthy Fats: About 11 grams
Fiber: About 6 grams
Notes: Avocado is a nutrient-dense source of monounsaturated fats.

Olive Oil:
Serving Size: 1 tablespoon
Calories: Approximately 120 calories
Healthy Fats: About 14 grams
Notes: Extra virgin olive oil is rich in monounsaturated fats and suitable for salad dressings or low-heat cooking.

Nuts (Almonds, Walnuts):
Serving Size: 1 ounce (about a handful)
Calories: Varies (e.g., almonds: around 160 calories)
Healthy Fats: About 14 grams (almonds)
Fiber: About 3.5 grams (almonds)
Notes: Nuts provide healthy fats, but portion control is key due to their calorie density.

Seeds (Chia Seeds, Flaxseeds):
Serving Size: 1 ounce
Calories: Varies (e.g., chia seeds: around 138 calories)
Healthy Fats: About 9 grams (chia seeds)
Fiber: About 10 grams (chia seeds)
Notes: Seeds are rich in omega-3 fatty acids and fiber.
Fatty Fish (Salmon, Mackerel):
Serving Size: 3 ounces cooked
Calories: Varies (e.g., salmon: around 155 calories)
Healthy Fats: About 8 grams (salmon)
Notes: Fatty fish provide omega-3 fatty acids, supporting heart health.

Coconut Oil:
Serving Size: 1 tablespoon
Calories: Approximately 120 calories
Healthy Fats: About 14 grams
Notes: Coconut oil is high in saturated fats; use in moderation.

Dark Chocolate (70-90% Cocoa):
Serving Size: 1 ounce
Calories: Approximately 150 calories
Healthy Fats: About 9 grams
Notes: Choose dark chocolate for a source of antioxidants and healthy fats.

Flaxseed Oil:
Serving Size: 1 tablespoon
Calories: Approximately 120 calories
Healthy Fats: About 14 grams
Notes: Flaxseed oil is a plant-based source of omega-3 fatty acids.

Cheese (Feta, Goat Cheese):
Serving Size: 1 ounce
Calories: Varies (e.g., feta: around 70 calories)
Healthy Fats: Varies (e.g., feta: about 6 grams)
Notes: Choose lower-fat cheese options in moderation.

Soybeans (Edamame):
Serving Size: 1 cup cooked
Calories: Approximately 190 calories
Healthy Fats: About 9 grams
Fiber: About 8 grams

Notes: Edamame is a plant-based source of healthy fats and protein.

Whole grains

Quinoa:
Serving Size: 1 cup cooked
Calories: Approximately 220 calories
Fiber: About 5 grams
Fat: About 4 grams
Notes: Quinoa is a complete protein and rich in fiber.

Brown Rice:
Serving Size: 1 cup cooked
Calories: Approximately 215 calories
Fiber: About 4 grams
Fat: 1.6 grams
Notes: Brown rice is a whole grain with higher fiber content than white rice.

Oats:
Serving Size: 1 cup cooked
Calories: Approximately 150 calories
Fiber: About 4 grams
Fat: 2.5 grams
Notes: Oats are high in soluble fiber, promoting digestive health.

Whole Wheat Pasta:
Serving Size: 1 cup cooked
Calories: Approximately 175 calories
Fiber: About 3.5 grams
Fat: 1.5 grams

Notes: Choose whole wheat for added fiber compared to refined pasta.

Barley:
Serving Size: 1 cup cooked
Calories: Approximately 193 calories
Fiber: About 6 grams
Fat: 0.7 grams
Notes: Barley provides both soluble and insoluble fiber.

Buckwheat:
Serving Size: 1 cup cooked
Calories: Approximately 155 calories
Fiber: About 4.5 grams
Fat: 1 gram
Notes: Buckwheat is gluten-free and a good source of nutrients.

Farro:
Serving Size: 1 cup cooked
Calories: Approximately 200 calories
Fiber: About 3.5 grams
Fat: 1 gram
Notes: Farro has a nutty flavor and is rich in fiber.

Millet:
Serving Size: 1 cup cooked
Calories: Approximately 207 calories
Fiber: About 2.3 grams
Fat: 1.7 grams
Notes: Millet is gluten-free and easy to digest.

Whole Wheat Bread:
Serving Size: 1 slice
Calories: Approximately 70-80 calories (varies)
Fiber: About 2-3 grams
Fat: 1-1.5 grams (varies)
Notes: Choose whole wheat for added fiber compared to white bread.

Amaranth:
Serving Size: 1 cup cooked
Calories: Approximately 250 calories
Fiber: About 5 grams
Fat: 3.5 grams
Notes: Amaranth is a gluten-free whole grain with a unique nutritional profile.

Low-fat dairy products

Low-Fat Greek Yogurt:
Serving Size: 1 cup
Calories: Approximately 100 calories
Fat: About 0.4 grams
Protein: About 20 grams
Notes: Greek yogurt is a rich source of protein with minimal fat.

Skim Milk:
Serving Size: 1 cup
Calories: Approximately 80 calories
Fat: 0 grams
Protein: About 8 grams
Notes: Skim milk is fat-free and provides calcium and vitamin D.

Low-Fat Cottage Cheese:
Serving Size: 1/2 cup
Calories: Approximately 80 calories
Fat: About 1 gram
Protein: About 14 grams
Notes: Cottage cheese is a protein-rich dairy option with minimal fat.

Low-Fat String Cheese:
Serving Size: 1 piece
Calories: Approximately 50 calories
Fat: About 1.5 grams
Protein: About 7 grams
Notes: String cheese is a convenient and portion-controlled snack.

Low-Fat Mozzarella Cheese:
Serving Size: 1 ounce
Calories: Approximately 70 calories
Fat: About 4.5 grams
Protein: About 7 grams
Notes: Mozzarella cheese adds flavor to dishes with moderate fat content.

Low-Fat Ricotta Cheese:
Serving Size: 1/2 cup
Calories: Approximately 180 calories
Fat: About 10 grams
Protein: About 14 grams
Notes: Use low-fat ricotta in recipes for added creaminess.

Low-Fat Sour Cream:
Serving Size: 2 tablespoons
Calories: Approximately 40 calories
Fat: About 2 grams
Protein: About 1 gram
Notes: Low-fat sour cream is a lighter alternative for dishes.

Low-Fat Yogurt Smoothie:
Serving Size: 1 bottle (varies)
Calories: Approximately 150-200 calories (varies)
Fat: Varies (typically low)
Protein: About 8-10 grams
Notes: Check labels for added sugars; choose options with minimal fat.

Low-Fat Swiss Cheese:
Serving Size: 1 ounce
Calories: Approximately 50 calories
Fat: About 2.5 grams
Protein: About 8 grams
Notes: Swiss cheese adds a mild flavor with lower fat content.

Low-Fat Buttermilk:
Serving Size: 1 cup
Calories: Approximately 100 calories
Fat: About 2 grams
Protein: About 8 grams
Notes: Buttermilk is a lower-fat option for cooking and baking

Spices and herbs

Turmeric:
Serving Size: Varies (often used in small amounts)
Calories: Negligible
Fat: Negligible
Fiber: Negligible
Notes: Turmeric has anti-inflammatory properties and is commonly used in savory dishes.

Ginger:
Serving Size: Varies (often used in small amounts)
Calories: Negligible
Fat: Negligible
Fiber: Negligible
Notes: Ginger is known for its digestive benefits and can be used in both sweet and savory dishes.

Cinnamon:
Serving Size: Varies (commonly used in small amounts)
Calories: Negligible
Fat: Negligible
Fiber: Negligible
Notes: Cinnamon adds a warm, sweet flavor and is often used in desserts and breakfast dishes.

Basil:
Serving Size: Varies (commonly used in small amounts)
Calories: Negligible
Fat: Negligible
Fiber: Negligible
Notes: Basil is a versatile herb that pairs well with a variety of dishes, both savory and sweet.

Cilantro (Coriander):
Serving Size: Varies (commonly used in small amounts)
Calories: Negligible
Fat: Negligible
Fiber: Negligible
Notes: Cilantro adds a fresh, citrusy flavor and is often used in Mexican and Asian cuisines.

Rosemary:
Serving Size: Varies (commonly used in small amounts)
Calories: Negligible
Fat: Negligible
Fiber: Negligible
Notes: Rosemary has a robust flavor and pairs well with roasted meats and vegetables.

Oregano:
Serving Size: Varies (commonly used in small amounts)
Calories: Negligible
Fat: Negligible
Fiber: Negligible
Notes: Oregano is commonly used in Mediterranean dishes, imparting a savory flavor.

Thyme:
Serving Size: Varies (commonly used in small amounts)
Calories: Negligible
Fat: Negligible
Fiber: Negligible

Notes: Thyme adds earthiness and is often used in soups, stews, and roasts.

Garlic:
Serving Size: Varies (commonly used in small amounts)
Calories: Negligible
Fat: Negligible
Fiber: Negligible
Notes: Garlic adds a pungent flavor and is a staple in various cuisines.

Parsley:
Serving Size: Varies (commonly used in small amounts)
Calories: Negligible
Fat: Negligible
Fiber: Negligible
Notes: Parsley adds a bright, fresh flavor and is often used as a garnish.

Beverages

Water:
Serving Size: Varies (8 cups or more recommended per day)
Calories: 0
Fat: 0 grams
Fiber: 0 grams
Notes: Staying hydrated is crucial for overall health and digestion. Aim for at least 8 cups of water daily.

Herbal Tea:
Serving Size: 1 tea bag or 1 teaspoon loose leaves

Calories: 0
Fat: 0 grams
Fiber: 0 grams
Notes: Herbal teas, such as chamomile or peppermint, can be soothing and aid in digestion.

Green Tea:
Serving Size: 1 tea bag or 1 teaspoon loose leaves
Calories: 0
Fat: 0 grams
Fiber: 0 grams
Notes: Green tea contains antioxidants and is low in calories.

Ginger Tea:
Serving Size: 1 tea bag or 1 teaspoon grated ginger
Calories: 0
Fat: 0 grams
Fiber: 0 grams
Notes: Ginger tea may help alleviate nausea and support digestion.

Vegetable Juice:
Serving Size: 1 cup
Calories: Varies (depending on vegetables used)
Fat: Varies (minimal)
Fiber: Varies (depending on vegetables used)
Notes: Fresh vegetable juices can provide nutrients without excessive calories or fat.

Coconut Water:
Serving Size: 1 cup
Calories: Approximately 46 calories
Fat: 0.5 grams
Fiber: 2 grams
Notes: Coconut water is a hydrating option with natural electrolytes.

Low-Fat Milk (Skim or 1%):
Serving Size: 1 cup
Calories: Approximately 80-100 calories (varies)
Fat: 0-2 grams (varies)
Fiber: 0 grams
Notes: Low-fat milk provides calcium and vitamin D with reduced fat content.

Almond Milk (Unsweetened):
Serving Size: 1 cup
Calories: Approximately 30-40 calories (varies)
Fat: 2.5-3 grams (varies)
Fiber: 1-2 grams (varies)
Notes: Unsweetened almond milk is a low-calorie dairy alternative.

Water with Lemon:
Serving Size: 1 cup
Calories: 0
Fat: 0 grams
Fiber: 0 grams
Notes: Lemon water can be refreshing and may aid digestion.

Chamomile Infusion:
Serving Size: 1 cup
Calories: 0
Fat: 0 grams
Fiber: 0 grams
Notes: Chamomile infusions can have calming effects and may support digestive health.

Snacks and sweets

Apple Slices with Almond Butter:
Serving Size: 1 medium apple with 1 tablespoon almond butter
Calories: Approximately 150 calories
Fat: About 7 grams
Fiber: About 4 grams
Notes: This snack provides a mix of fiber, healthy fats, and natural sweetness.

Greek Yogurt Parfait:
Serving Size: 1 cup low-fat Greek yogurt with berries and a sprinkle of granola
Calories: Approximately 200-250 calories (varies)
Fat: About 3-5 grams (varies)
Fiber: About 4-6 grams (varies)
Notes: Greek yogurt offers protein, while berries and granola add fiber and natural sweetness.

Dark Chocolate-Covered Almonds:
Serving Size: 1 ounce (about 23 almonds)
Calories: Approximately 160 calories
Fat: About 13 grams
Fiber: About 3 grams

Notes: Dark chocolate provides antioxidants, and almonds offer healthy fats.

Hummus with Vegetable Sticks:
Serving Size: 2 tablespoons hummus with carrot and cucumber sticks
Calories: Approximately 100 calories
Fat: About 6 grams
Fiber: About 3 grams
Notes: Hummus provides protein, and vegetables add fiber and crunch.

Air-Popped Popcorn:
Serving Size: 3 cups
Calories: Approximately 90 calories
Fat: About 1 gram
Fiber: About 3.5 grams
Notes: Popcorn is a whole grain snack with minimal fat.

Frozen Grapes:
Serving Size: 1 cup
Calories: Approximately 60 calories
Fat: 0 grams
Fiber: About 1 gram
Notes: Frozen grapes offer a sweet and refreshing treat.

Cottage Cheese with Pineapple:
Serving Size: 1/2 cup low-fat cottage cheese with 1/2 cup pineapple chunks
Calories: Approximately 120 calories
Fat: About 1 gram

Fiber: About 1.5 grams
Notes: Cottage cheese provides protein, and pineapple adds natural sweetness.

Rice Cakes with Avocado:
Serving Size: 2 rice cakes with 1/2 avocado
Calories: Approximately 200 calories
Fat: About 12 grams
Fiber: About 5 grams
Notes: This snack combines whole grains with healthy fats.

Trail Mix:
Serving Size: 1/4 cup
Calories: Approximately 150 calories
Fat: About 10 grams
Fiber: About 2 grams
Notes: Choose a mix with nuts, seeds, and dried fruit for variety.

Smoothie Bowl:
Serving Size: 1 cup blended smoothie topped with berries and a sprinkle of nuts
Calories: Approximately 200-250 calories (varies)
Fat: About 5-8 grams (varies)
Fiber: About 4-6 grams (varies)
Notes: Use ingredients like yogurt, fruits, and nuts for a nutrient-rich snack.

General Recommendations:

Daily Fat Intake: Aim to limit total daily fat intake, with a focus on healthy fats. The American Heart

Association suggests 20-35% of total daily calories from fat, emphasizing monounsaturated and polyunsaturated fats.

Serving Size Consideration: Start with small servings and monitor your body's responses. Gradually increase portion sizes as tolerated.

Individual Tolerances: Individual responses to vegetables can vary, so pay attention to your body's reactions and modify your diet according

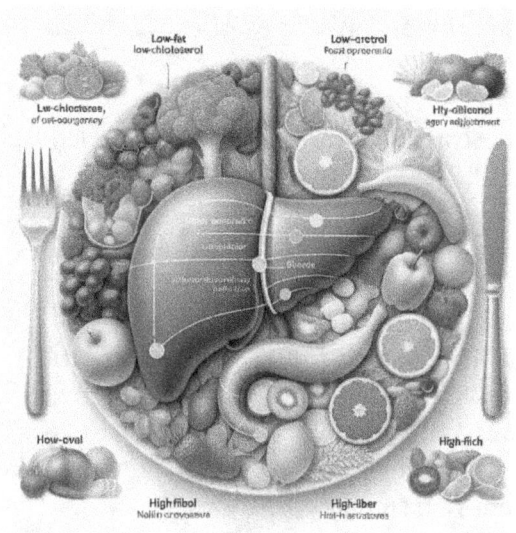

PART 3

HEALTHY SAMPLE MEAL PLANS AND RECIPES

Breakfast ideas

1. Greek Yogurt Parfait:
Ingredients:
1 cup low-fat Greek yogurt
1/2 cup fresh berries
1/4 cup granola

Preparation:
Layer Greek yogurt, berries, and granola in a glass or bowl.
Nutritional Information:
Calories: Approximately 250 calories
Fat: About 6 grams
Fiber: About 4 grams

2. Oatmeal with Almond Butter and Banana:
Ingredients:
1/2 cup rolled oats
1 cup water or milk
1 tablespoon almond butter
1/2 banana, sliced

Preparation:
Cook oats with water or milk, top with almond butter and banana slices.
Nutritional Information:

Calories: Approximately 300 calories
Fat: About 11 grams
Fiber: About 7 grams

3. Egg and Vegetable Scramble:
Ingredients:
2 eggs, scrambled
1/2 cup diced bell peppers and tomatoes
1 tablespoon olive oil
Preparation:
Sauté vegetables in olive oil, add scrambled eggs, cook until done.
Nutritional Information:
Calories: Approximately 250 calories
Fat: About 18 grams
Fiber: About 3 grams

4. Smoothie Bowl:
Ingredients:
1 cup blended fruit smoothie (e.g., banana, berries, yogurt)
2 tablespoons granola
1 tablespoon chia seeds

Preparation:
Pour smoothie into a bowl, top with granola and chia seeds.
Nutritional Information:
Calories: Approximately 200-250 calories
Fat: About 5-8 grams
Fiber: About 4-6 grams

5. Whole Wheat Toast with Avocado:
Ingredients:
2 slices whole wheat toast
1/2 avocado, mashed
Salt and pepper to taste

Preparation:
Toast bread, spread mashed avocado, season with salt and pepper.
Nutritional Information:
Calories: Approximately 250 calories
Fat: About 15 grams
Fiber: About 7 grams

6. Cottage Cheese and Pineapple Bowl:
Ingredients:
1/2 cup low-fat cottage cheese
1/2 cup fresh pineapple chunks
1 tablespoon chopped nuts

Preparation:
Combine cottage cheese, pineapple, and sprinkle with chopped nuts.
Nutritional Information:
Calories: Approximately 220 calories
Fat: About 5 grams
Fiber: About 1.5 grams

7. Chia Seed Pudding:
Ingredients:
3 tablespoons chia seeds
1 cup almond milk (unsweetened)
1/2 teaspoon vanilla extract

1 tablespoon honey

Preparation:
Mix all ingredients, refrigerate overnight, and top with berries.
Nutritional Information:
Calories: Approximately 180 calories
Fat: About 8 grams
Fiber: About 10 grams

8. Quinoa Breakfast Bowl:
Ingredients:
1/2 cup cooked quinoa
1/4 cup Greek yogurt
1/4 cup mixed berries
1 tablespoon honey

Preparation:
Combine quinoa, Greek yogurt, and top with berries and honey.
Nutritional Information:
Calories: Approximately 250 calories
Fat: About 5 grams
Fiber: About 4 grams

9. Whole Grain Pancakes with Berries:
Ingredients:
2 whole grain pancakes
1/2 cup mixed berries
1 tablespoon maple syrup

Preparation:
Prepare pancakes, top with berries, and drizzle with maple syrup.
Nutritional Information:
Calories: Approximately 300 calories
Fat: About 4 grams
Fiber: About 5 grams

10. Vegetarian Breakfast Burrito:
Ingredients:
1 whole wheat tortilla
2 scrambled eggs
1/4 cup black beans, drained and rinsed
Salsa and avocado slices

Preparation:
Fill the tortilla with scrambled eggs, black beans, salsa, and avocado.
Nutritional Information:
Calories: Approximately 300 calories
Fat: About 12 grams
Fiber: About 8 grams

Lunch suggestions

1. Grilled Chicken Salad:
Ingredients:
4 oz grilled chicken breast
Mixed greens
Cherry tomatoes, sliced cucumber
Olive oil and lemon dressing

Preparation:
Grill chicken, toss with vegetables, and drizzle with dressing.
Nutritional Information:
Calories: Approximately 300 calories
Fat: About 15 grams
Fiber: About 4 grams

2. Quinoa and Vegetable Bowl:
Ingredients:
1/2 cup cooked quinoa
Roasted vegetables (e.g., bell peppers, zucchini)
Feta cheese
Lemon-tahini dressing

Preparation:
Combine quinoa, roasted vegetables, and top with feta and dressing.
Nutritional Information:
Calories: Approximately 350 calories
Fat: About 15 grams
Fiber: About 8 grams

3. Salmon and Asparagus Packets:
Ingredients:
4 oz baked salmon
Asparagus spears
Lemon slices, dill, salt, and pepper

Preparation:
Place salmon and asparagus in foil, season, bake until cooked.
Nutritional Information:
Calories: Approximately 300 calories
Fat: About 15 grams
Fiber: About 3 grams

4. Mediterranean Chickpea Salad:
Ingredients:
1 cup canned chickpeas (drained)
Cherry tomatoes, cucumber, red onion
Feta cheese, olives
Olive oil and balsamic vinegar dressing

Preparation:
Mix all ingredients and toss with dressing.
Nutritional Information:
Calories: Approximately 250 calories
Fat: About 10 grams
Fiber: About 7 grams

5. Vegetable Stir-Fry with Tofu:
Ingredients:
1 cup tofu cubes
Mixed stir-fry vegetables (broccoli, bell peppers, snap peas)

Soy sauce, ginger, garlic

Preparation:
Sauté tofu and vegetables with soy sauce, ginger, and garlic.
Nutritional Information:
Calories: Approximately 300 calories
Fat: About 12 grams
Fiber: About 6 grams

6. Turkey and Avocado Wrap:
Ingredients:
4 oz deli turkey slices
Whole grain wrap
Avocado slices, lettuce, tomato
Mustard or Greek yogurt dressing

Preparation:
Assemble ingredients in a wrap.
Nutritional Information:
Calories: Approximately 350 calories
Fat: About 15 grams
Fiber: About 7 grams

7. Whole Wheat Pasta with Pesto and Cherry Tomatoes:
Ingredients:
1 cup whole wheat pasta
Homemade or store-bought pesto
Cherry tomatoes, Parmesan cheese

Preparation:
Cook pasta, toss with pesto, add cherry tomatoes and cheese.
Nutritional Information:
Calories: Approximately 400 calories
Fat: About 18 grams
Fiber: About 5 grams

8. Vegetarian Bean Burrito Bowl:
Ingredients:
1/2 cup cooked black beans
Brown rice
Sautéed peppers and onions
Guacamole, salsa, Greek yogurt

Preparation:
Layer beans, rice, vegetables, and toppings.
Nutritional Information:
Calories: Approximately 350 calories
Fat: About 12 grams
Fiber: About 8 grams

9. Shrimp and Quinoa Salad:
Ingredients:
4 oz grilled shrimp
Quinoa, cooked
Spinach, cherry tomatoes, red onion
Lemon vinaigrette dressing

Preparation:
Combine ingredients, drizzle with dressing.
Nutritional Information:
Calories: Approximately 300 calories

Fat: About 10 grams
Fiber: About 5 grams

10. Egg Salad Lettuce Wraps:
Ingredients:
2 hard-boiled eggs, chopped
Greek yogurt
Lettuce leaves
Dijon mustard, salt, and pepper

Preparation:
Mix eggs with Greek yogurt and seasonings, serve in lettuce wraps.
Nutritional Information:
Calories: Approximately 250 calories
Fat: About 12 grams
Fiber: About 3 grams

Dinner options

1. Baked Lemon Herb Chicken:
Ingredients:
6 oz boneless, skinless chicken breast
Lemon juice, garlic, rosemary, thyme

Preparation:
Marinate chicken in lemon juice, garlic, and herbs, bake until cooked.
Nutritional Information:
Calories: Approximately 250 calories
Fat: About 8 grams
Fiber: About 0 grams

2. Quinoa Stuffed Bell Peppers:
Ingredients:
1 cup cooked quinoa
Ground turkey or lean beef
Bell peppers, tomato sauce

Preparation:
Mix quinoa, cooked meat, and stuff into bell peppers, bake.
Nutritional Information:
Calories: Approximately 300 calories
Fat: About 10 grams
Fiber: About 5 grams

3. Salmon with Roasted Vegetables:
Ingredients:
6 oz baked or grilled salmon
Mixed roasted vegetables (e.g., broccoli, carrots)

Preparation:
Season salmon, bake or grill, serve with roasted veggies.
Nutritional Information:
Calories: Approximately 350 calories
Fat: About 18 grams
Fiber: About 5 grams

4. Vegetable and Lentil Soup:
Ingredients:
Mixed vegetables (carrots, celery, kale)
Lentils, low-sodium broth
Herbs and spices

Preparation:
Simmer vegetables, lentils, and seasonings in broth.
Nutritional Information:
Calories: Approximately 200 calories
Fat: About 3 grams
Fiber: About 8 grams

5. Grilled Shrimp Salad:
Ingredients:
4 oz grilled shrimp
Mixed greens, cherry tomatoes, cucumber
Olive oil and balsamic dressing

Preparation:
Grill shrimp, toss with greens and dressing.
Nutritional Information:
Calories: Approximately 250 calories
Fat: About 12 grams
Fiber: About 3 grams

6. Stir-Fried Tofu with Broccoli:
Ingredients:
1 cup tofu cubes
Broccoli florets, bell peppers
Low-sodium soy sauce, ginger, garlic

Preparation:
Sauté tofu and vegetables with soy sauce, ginger, and garlic.
Nutritional Information:
Calories: Approximately 300 calories
Fat: About 15 grams
Fiber: About 5 grams

7. Vegetarian Quinoa Bowl:
Ingredients:
1 cup cooked quinoa
Black beans, corn, diced tomatoes
Avocado slices, cilantro, lime

Preparation:
Mix quinoa with beans, corn, tomatoes, top with avocado and cilantro.
Nutritional Information:
Calories: Approximately 350 calories
Fat: About 15 grams
Fiber: About 10 grams

8. Turkey and Vegetable Skewers:
Ingredients:
4 oz turkey breast cubes
Bell peppers, cherry tomatoes, zucchini

Preparation:
Thread turkey and vegetables onto skewers, grill or bake.
Nutritional Information:
Calories: Approximately 300 calories
Fat: About 8 grams
Fiber: About 4 grams

9. Baked Cod with Lemon and Herbs:
Ingredients:
6 oz cod fillet
Lemon, parsley, dill

Preparation:
Season cod with lemon and herbs, bake until flaky.
Nutritional Information:
Calories: Approximately 200 calories
Fat: About 5 grams
Fiber: About 0 grams

10. Vegetable and Chicken Sauté:
Ingredients:
4 oz grilled chicken breast
Mixed vegetables (asparagus, cherry tomatoes, bell peppers)
Olive oil, garlic, herbs

Preparation:
Sauté chicken and vegetables in olive oil with garlic and herbs.
Nutritional Information:
Calories: Approximately 350 calories
Fat: About 15 grams

Fiber: About 5 grams

Healthy snack recipes

1. Almond Butter and Banana Rice Cakes:
Ingredients:
Rice cakes
Almond butter
Sliced bananas

Preparation:
Spread almond butter on rice cakes and top with banana slices.
Nutritional Information:
Calories: Approximately 200 calories
Fat: About 10 grams
Fiber: About 3 grams

2. Greek Yogurt Parfait with Berries:
Ingredients:
Low-fat Greek yogurt
Mixed berries (strawberries, blueberries)
Granola

Preparation:
Layer yogurt, berries, and granola in a glass or bowl.
Nutritional Information:
Calories: Approximately 250 calories
Fat: About 5 grams
Fiber: About 4 grams

3. Hummus and Veggie Sticks:
Ingredients:
Hummus

Carrot and cucumber sticks

Preparation:
Dip vegetable sticks into hummus.
Nutritional Information:
Calories: Approximately 150 calories
Fat: About 8 grams
Fiber: About 4 grams

4. Baked Apple Chips:
Ingredients:
Apples, thinly sliced
Cinnamon

Preparation:
Toss apple slices with cinnamon, bake until crispy.
Nutritional Information:
Calories: Approximately 100 calories
Fat: About 0.5 grams
Fiber: About 4 grams

5. Cottage Cheese with Pineapple:
Ingredients:
Low-fat cottage cheese
Pineapple chunks

Preparation:
Mix cottage cheese with pineapple.
Nutritional Information:
Calories: Approximately 150 calories
Fat: About 2 grams
Fiber: About 1.5 grams

6. Whole Grain Crackers with Tuna Salad:
Ingredients:
Whole grain crackers
Canned tuna, drained
Greek yogurt, celery, and onion

Preparation:
Mix tuna with Greek yogurt, celery, and onion, serve
on crackers.
Nutritional Information:
Calories: Approximately 200 calories
Fat: About 5 grams
Fiber: About 3 grams

7. Mixed Nuts and Dried Fruit Trail Mix:
Ingredients:
Mixed nuts (almonds, walnuts, pistachios)
Dried fruit (apricots, cranberries)

Preparation:
Combine nuts and dried fruit for a trail mix.
Nutritional Information:
Calories: Approximately 200 calories
Fat: About 15 grams
Fiber: About 3 grams

8. Avocado and Tomato Salsa on Whole Grain Toast:
Ingredients:
Whole grain toast
Avocado slices
Diced tomatoes, cilantro, lime

Preparation:

Spread avocado on toast, top with tomato salsa.
Nutritional Information:
Calories: Approximately 250 calories
Fat: About 12 grams
Fiber: About 5 grams

9. Chia Seed Pudding:
Ingredients:
Chia seeds
Almond milk
Vanilla extract, honey

Preparation:
Mix chia seeds with almond milk, vanilla, and honey,
refrigerate until thick.
Nutritional Information:
Calories: Approximately 150 calories
Fat: About 7 grams
Fiber: About 10 grams

10. Yogurt-Dipped Strawberries:
Ingredients:
Strawberries
Greek yogurt

Preparation:
Dip strawberries in Greek yogurt, freeze until firm.
Nutritional Information:
Calories: Approximately 100 calories
Fat: About 2 grams
Fiber: About 3 grams

Smoothies

1. Berry Blast Smoothie:
Ingredients:
1 cup mixed berries (strawberries, blueberries, raspberries)
1/2 banana
1/2 cup low-fat Greek yogurt
1/2 cup almond milk (unsweetened)

Preparation:
Blend all ingredients until smooth.
Nutritional Information:
Calories: Approximately 150 calories
Fat: About 3 grams
Fiber: About 5 grams

2. Green Goddess Smoothie:
Ingredients:
1 cup spinach
1/2 cucumber
1/2 avocado
1/2 cup pineapple chunks
1 cup coconut water

Preparation:
Blend all ingredients until smooth.
Nutritional Information:
Calories: Approximately 200 calories
Fat: About 10 grams
Fiber: About 7 grams

3. Banana-Oat Power Smoothie:
Ingredients:
1 banana
1/4 cup rolled oats
1 tablespoon almond butter
1 cup skim milk

Preparation:
Blend all ingredients until smooth.
Nutritional Information:
Calories: Approximately 250 calories
Fat: About 8 grams
Fiber: About 4 grams

4. Tropical Paradise Smoothie:
Ingredients:
1/2 cup mango chunks
1/2 cup pineapple chunks
1/2 banana
1/2 cup coconut water

Preparation:
Blend all ingredients until smooth.
Nutritional Information:
Calories: Approximately 180 calories
Fat: About 2 grams
Fiber: About 3 grams

5. Protein-Packed Almond Joy Smoothie:
Ingredients:
1 scoop protein powder (whey or plant-based)
1 tablespoon unsweetened cocoa powder
1 tablespoon almond butter

1/2 banana
1 cup almond milk (unsweetened)

Preparation:
Blend all ingredients until smooth.
Nutritional Information:
Calories: Approximately 300 calories
Fat: About 15 grams
Fiber: About 6 grams

6. Peachy Keen Chia Smoothie:
Ingredients:
1 cup sliced peaches (fresh or frozen)
1 tablespoon chia seeds
1/2 cup low-fat Greek yogurt
1 cup water or almond milk

Preparation:
Blend all ingredients until smooth.
Nutritional Information:
Calories: Approximately 200 calories
Fat: About 6 grams
Fiber: About 6 grams

7. Citrus Burst Immunity Smoothie:
Ingredients:
1/2 orange, peeled
1/2 grapefruit, peeled
1/2 banana
1/2 cup low-fat plain yogurt
1/2 cup water or coconut water

Preparation:
Blend all ingredients until smooth.
Nutritional Information:
Calories: Approximately 160 calories
Fat: About 2 grams
Fiber: About 4 grams

8. Strawberry Kiwi Antioxidant Smoothie:
Ingredients:
1 cup strawberries
2 kiwis, peeled
1/2 banana
1/2 cup coconut water

Preparation:
Blend all ingredients until smooth.
Nutritional Information:
Calories: Approximately 150 calories
Fat: About 2 grams
Fiber: About 5 grams

9. Vanilla Almond Chai Smoothie:
Ingredients:
1 cup unsweetened vanilla almond milk
1/2 banana
1/2 teaspoon chai spice blend
1 scoop vanilla protein powder

Preparation:
Blend all ingredients until smooth.
Nutritional Information:
Calories: Approximately 200 calories
Fat: About 7 grams

Fiber: About 4 grams

10. Blueberry Almond Butter Smoothie Bowl:
Ingredients:
1/2 cup blueberries
1 tablespoon almond butter
1/2 banana
1/4 cup granola
1/4 cup low-fat Greek yogurt

Preparation:
Blend blueberries, almond butter, and bananas. Pour into a bowl, top with granola and yogurt.
Nutritional Information:
Calories: Approximately 250 calories
Fat: About 8 grams
Fiber: About 6 grams

Desserts

1. Frozen Banana Bites:
Ingredients:
Bananas, sliced
Dark chocolate, melted
Chopped nuts or shredded coconut (optional)

Preparation:
Dip banana slices in melted dark chocolate, sprinkle with nuts or coconut, and freeze.
Nutritional Information:
Calories: Approximately 100 calories per serving
Fat: About 5 grams
Fiber: About 2 grams

2. Chia Seed Pudding with Berries:
Ingredients:
Chia seeds
Almond milk
Mixed berries
Honey or maple syrup for sweetness

Preparation:
Mix chia seeds with almond milk, add berries, and refrigerate until thickened.
Nutritional Information:
Calories: Approximately 150 calories per serving
Fat: About 5 grams
Fiber: About 8 grams

3. Greek Yogurt Parfait with Nuts and Honey:
Ingredients:
Low-fat Greek yogurt
Mixed nuts (almonds, walnuts)
Honey

Preparation:
Layer yogurt, nuts, and drizzle with honey.
Nutritional Information:
Calories: Approximately 200 calories per serving
Fat: About 10 grams
Fiber: About 2 grams

4. Baked Apples with Cinnamon:
Ingredients:
Apples, cored and sliced
Cinnamon
Greek yogurt (optional)

Preparation:
Sprinkle apple slices with cinnamon and bake until tender. Serve with a dollop of Greek yogurt if desired.
Nutritional Information:
Calories: Approximately 100 calories per serving
Fat: About 1 gram
Fiber: About 3 grams

5. Dark Chocolate-Covered Strawberries:
Ingredients:
Strawberries, washed and dried
Dark chocolate, melted

Preparation:
Dip strawberries in melted dark chocolate and let them set.
Nutritional Information:
Calories: Approximately 50 calories per strawberry
Fat: About 2 grams
Fiber: About 2 grams

6. Coconut Mango Rice Pudding:
Ingredients:
Cooked brown rice
Coconut milk
Diced mango
Coconut flakes

Preparation:
Mix rice with coconut milk, top with mango and coconut flakes.
Nutritional Information:

Calories: Approximately 200 calories per serving
Fat: About 8 grams
Fiber: About 3 grams

7. Frozen Yogurt Bark with Berries:
Ingredients:
Low-fat Greek yogurt
Mixed berries
Honey for sweetness

Preparation:
Spread yogurt on a parchment-lined tray, top with berries, and drizzle with honey. Freeze and break into pieces.
Nutritional Information:
Calories: Approximately 100 calories per serving
Fat: About 3 grams
Fiber: About 2 grams

8. Pumpkin Chia Seed Pudding:
Ingredients:
Canned pumpkin puree
Chia seeds
Pumpkin pie spice
Maple syrup for sweetness

Preparation:
Mix pumpkin puree, chia seeds, spice, and sweeten with maple syrup. Refrigerate until thickened.
Nutritional Information:
Calories: Approximately 150 calories per serving
Fat: About 6 grams
Fiber: About 8 grams

9. Fruit Salad with Mint-Lime Dressing:
Ingredients:
Mixed fruits (e.g., melon, berries, kiwi)
Fresh mint leaves
Lime juice

Preparation:
Toss fruits with mint and lime dressing.
Nutritional Information:
Calories: Approximately 80 calories per serving
Fat: About 0.5 grams
Fiber: About 2 grams

10. Avocado Chocolate Mousse:
Ingredients:
Ripe avocados
Unsweetened cocoa powder
Maple syrup or honey for sweetness

Preparation:
Blend avocados, cocoa powder, and sweetener until smooth.
Nutritional Information:
Calories: Approximately 150 calories per serving
Fat: About 10 grams
Fiber: About 5 grams

BONUS: 45-DAYS MEAL PLAN

Day 1: Grilled Lemon Herb Chicken
Ingredients:
6 oz boneless, skinless chicken breast
Lemon juice, garlic, rosemary, thyme

Preparation:
Marinate chicken in lemon juice, garlic, and herbs, grill until cooked.
Nutritional Information:
Calories: Approximately 250 calories
Fat: About 8 grams
Fiber: About 0 grams

Day 2: Quinoa and Vegetable Stir-Fry
Ingredients:
1 cup cooked quinoa
Mixed stir-fry vegetables (broccoli, bell peppers, snap peas)
Low-sodium soy sauce, ginger, garlic

Preparation:
Sauté vegetables and mix with cooked quinoa and soy sauce.
Nutritional Information:
Calories: Approximately 300 calories
Fat: About 12 grams
Fiber: About 6 grams

Day 3: Greek Yogurt and Berry Parfait
Ingredients:
Low-fat Greek yogurt
Mixed berries (strawberries, blueberries)

Granola

Preparation:
Layer yogurt, berries, and granola in a glass or bowl.
Nutritional Information:
Calories: Approximately 250 calories
Fat: About 5 grams
Fiber: About 4 grams

Day 4: Baked Cod with Lemon and Herbs
Ingredients:
6 oz cod fillet
Lemon, parsley, dill

Preparation:
Season cod with lemon and herbs, bake until flaky.
Nutritional Information:
Calories: Approximately 200 calories
Fat: About 5 grams
Fiber: About 0 grams

Day 5: Lentil and Vegetable Soup
Ingredients:
Mixed vegetables (carrots, celery, kale)
Lentils, low-sodium broth
Herbs and spices

Preparation:
Simmer vegetables, lentils, and seasonings in broth.
Nutritional Information:
Calories: Approximately 200 calories
Fat: About 3 grams
Fiber: About 8 grams

Day 6: Turkey and Quinoa Stuffed Bell Peppers
Ingredients:
1 cup cooked quinoa
Ground turkey or lean beef
Bell peppers, tomato sauce

Preparation:
Mix quinoa, cooked meat, and stuff into bell peppers, bake.
Nutritional Information:
Calories: Approximately 300 calories
Fat: About 10 grams
Fiber: About 5 grams

Day 7: Salmon and Asparagus Packets
Ingredients:
4 oz baked salmon
Asparagus spears
Lemon slices, dill, salt, and pepper

Preparation:
Place salmon and asparagus in foil, season, bake until cooked.
Nutritional Information:
Calories: Approximately 300 calories
Fat: About 15 grams
Fiber: About 3 grams

Day 8: Greek Salad with Grilled Chicken
Ingredients:
4 oz grilled chicken breast
Mixed greens, cucumber, cherry tomatoes, feta cheese, olives

Olive oil and balsamic vinegar dressing

Preparation:
Toss all ingredients with dressing.
Nutritional Information:
Calories: Approximately 300 calories
Fat: About 15 grams
Fiber: About 4 grams

Day 9: Quinoa and Black Bean Bowl
Ingredients:
1 cup cooked quinoa
Black beans, corn, diced tomatoes
Avocado slices, cilantro, lime

Preparation:
Mix quinoa with beans, corn, tomatoes, top with avocado and cilantro.
Nutritional Information:
Calories: Approximately 350 calories
Fat: About 15 grams
Fiber: About 10 grams

Day 10: Greek Yogurt Chicken Salad Lettuce Wraps
Ingredients:
4 oz cooked chicken breast, shredded
Low-fat Greek yogurt
Lettuce leaves, cucumber, tomato
Dijon mustard, salt, and pepper

Preparation:
Mix chicken with Greek yogurt, seasonings, and serve in lettuce wraps.

Nutritional Information:
Calories: Approximately 250 calories
Fat: About 12 grams
Fiber: About 3 grams

Day 11: Shrimp and Quinoa Salad
Ingredients:
4 oz grilled shrimp
Mixed greens, cherry tomatoes, cucumber
Olive oil and balsamic dressing

Preparation:
Grill shrimp, toss with greens and dressing.
Nutritional Information:
Calories: Approximately 250 calories
Fat: About 12 grams
Fiber: About 3 grams

Day 12: Veggie and Tofu Stir-Fry
Ingredients:
1 cup tofu cubes
Broccoli florets, bell peppers
Low-sodium soy sauce, ginger, garlic

Preparation:
Sauté tofu and vegetables with soy sauce, ginger, and
garlic.
Nutritional Information:
Calories: Approximately 300 calories
Fat: About 15 grams
Fiber: About 5 grams

Day 13: Baked Chicken Thighs with Herbs
Ingredients:
6 oz bone-in, skinless chicken thighs
Rosemary, thyme, garlic, lemon

Preparation:
Season chicken with herbs and bake until cooked.
Nutritional Information:
Calories: Approximately 250 calories
Fat: About 15 grams
Fiber: About 0 grams

Day 14: Quinoa Salad with Chickpeas
Ingredients:
1 cup cooked quinoa
Chickpeas, cucumber, cherry tomatoes, red onion
Lemon-tahini dressing

Preparation:
Mix quinoa and vegetables, drizzle with dressing.
Nutritional Information:
Calories: Approximately 300 calories
Fat: About 12 grams
Fiber: About 8 grams

Day 15: Turkey and Vegetable Skewers
Ingredients:
4 oz turkey breast cubes
Bell peppers, cherry tomatoes, zucchini

Preparation:
Thread turkey and vegetables onto skewers, grill or
bake.

Nutritional Information:
Calories: Approximately 300 calories
Fat: About 8 grams
Fiber: About 4 grams

Day 16: Grilled Swordfish with Mango Salsa
Ingredients:
6 oz grilled swordfish
Mango, red onion, cilantro, lime

Preparation:
Top grilled swordfish with mango salsa.
Nutritional Information:
Calories: Approximately 250 calories
Fat: About 10 grams
Fiber: About 2 grams

Day 17: Lentil and Spinach Stuffed Bell Peppers
Ingredients:
Cooked lentils
Spinach, bell peppers
Tomato sauce, Italian herbs

Preparation:
Mix lentils, spinach, and herbs, stuff into bell peppers, bake.
Nutritional Information:
Calories: Approximately 250 calories
Fat: About 5 grams
Fiber: About 8 grams

Day 18: Asian-Inspired Chicken Lettuce Wraps
Ingredients:
4 oz ground chicken
Water chestnuts, mushrooms, green onions
Soy sauce, hoisin sauce, ginger

Preparation:
Sauté chicken with vegetables and sauces, served in lettuce wraps.
Nutritional Information:
Calories: Approximately 250 calories
Fat: About 12 grams
Fiber: About 3 grams

Day 19: Quinoa and Avocado Salad
Ingredients:
1 cup cooked quinoa
Avocado, cherry tomatoes, cucumber
Lime vinaigrette

Preparation:
Mix quinoa and vegetables, toss with lime vinaigrette.
Nutritional Information:
Calories: Approximately 300 calories
Fat: About 15 grams
Fiber: About 6 grams

Day 20: Grilled Vegetable and Chicken Kabobs
Ingredients:
4 oz grilled chicken breast
Assorted vegetables (zucchini, bell peppers, cherry tomatoes)

Olive oil, garlic, herbs
Preparation:
Marinate chicken and vegetables, thread onto skewers, grill until cooked.
Nutritional Information:
Calories: Approximately 300 calories
Fat: About 10 grams
Fiber: About 5 grams

Day 21: Baked Tilapia with Mango Salsa
Ingredients:
6 oz baked tilapia
Mango, red onion, cilantro, lime

Preparation:
Top baked tilapia with mango salsa.
Nutritional Information:
Calories: Approximately 250 calories
Fat: About 8 grams
Fiber: About 2 grams

Day 22: Quinoa and Black Bean Stuffed Peppers
Ingredients:
1 cup cooked quinoa
Black beans, corn, diced tomatoes
Avocado slices, cilantro, lime

Preparation:
Mix quinoa with beans, corn, tomatoes, top with avocado and cilantro.
Nutritional Information:
Calories: Approximately 350 calories
Fat: About 15 grams

Fiber: About 10 grams

Day 23: Turkey and Vegetable Stir-Fry
Ingredients:
4 oz ground turkey
Mixed stir-fry vegetables (broccoli, bell peppers, snap peas)
Low-sodium soy sauce, ginger, garlic

Preparation:
Sauté turkey and mix with stir-fried vegetables and soy sauce.
Nutritional Information:
Calories: Approximately 300 calories
Fat: About 12 grams
Fiber: About 6 grams

Day 24: Chickpea and Spinach Curry
Ingredients:
Chickpeas, spinach, tomatoes
Onion, garlic, ginger, curry spices

Preparation:
Simmer chickpeas, spinach, and spices in tomato-based sauce.
Nutritional Information:
Calories: Approximately 250 calories
Fat: About 8 grams
Fiber: About 8 grams

Day 25: Greek Yogurt and Berry Smoothie Bowl
Ingredients:
Low-fat Greek yogurt

Mixed berries (strawberries, blueberries)
Granola, chia seeds

Preparation:
Blend yogurt and berries, pour into a bowl, top with granola and chia seeds.
Nutritional Information:
Calories: Approximately 250 calories
Fat: About 5 grams
Fiber: About 4 grams

Day 26: Lemon Herb Grilled Chicken Salad
Ingredients:
4 oz grilled chicken breast
Mixed greens, cherry tomatoes, cucumber
Lemon herb dressing

Preparation:
Grill chicken, toss with greens, and drizzle with lemon herb dressing.
Nutritional Information:
Calories: Approximately 250 calories
Fat: About 10 grams
Fiber: About 4 grams

Day 27: Quinoa and Vegetable Buddha Bowl
Ingredients:
1 cup cooked quinoa
Mixed roasted vegetables (sweet potatoes, Brussels sprouts, cauliflower)
Tahini dressing

Preparation:
Arrange quinoa and roasted vegetables in a bowl, drizzle with tahini dressing.
Nutritional Information:
Calories: Approximately 300 calories
Fat: About 15 grams
Fiber: About 8 grams

Day 28: Baked Cod with Mediterranean Salsa
Ingredients:
6 oz baked cod fillet
Tomatoes, olives, red onion, parsley, olive oil

Preparation:
Top baked cod with Mediterranean salsa.
Nutritional Information:
Calories: Approximately 250 calories
Fat: About 8 grams
Fiber: About 2 grams

Day 29: Lentil and Vegetable Stuffed Portobello Mushrooms
Ingredients:
Cooked lentils
Mixed vegetables (bell peppers, spinach)
Portobello mushrooms

Preparation:
Mix lentils and vegetables, stuff into portobello mushrooms, and bake.
Nutritional Information:
Calories: Approximately 250 calories
Fat: About 5 grams

Fiber: About 8 grams

Day 30: Grilled Chicken Caesar Salad
Ingredients:
4 oz grilled chicken breast
Romaine lettuce, cherry tomatoes, Parmesan cheese
Caesar dressing (light)

Preparation:
Grill chicken, toss with lettuce, tomatoes, and drizzle
with Caesar dressing.
Nutritional Information:
Calories: Approximately 300 calories
Fat: About 15 grams
Fiber: About 4 grams

CONCLUSION

In conclusion, the journey through a Gallbladder Diet After Removal is not just a dietary adjustment but a transformative experience that shapes one's path to recovery. As we've seen in John's story, the commitment to understanding the nuances of post-surgery nutrition and making conscious lifestyle adjustments can pave the way for a healthier and more fulfilling life.

The importance of immediate post-surgery diet guidelines, marked by clear liquids and broths, cannot be overstated. These choices create a gentle introduction to the world of foods after gallbladder removal, allowing the body to heal and adapt. Gradually reintroducing soft foods ensures a smooth transition, fostering a sense of comfort and aiding the recovery process.

Beyond the initial days, the Gallbladder Diet takes on a long-term dimension, emphasizing the incorporation of nutrient-rich foods into one's daily routine. Fruits, vegetables, lean proteins, and whole grains become not just dietary choices but companions in the journey toward overall well-being.

The impact of this dietary shift extends beyond the physical realm. It speaks to a commitment to one's health, resilience in the face of change, and an appreciation for the intricacies of the human body. Through ongoing communication with healthcare providers, a proactive approach to kitchen preparation, and a conscious selection of foods, individuals can navigate the post-gallbladder removal landscape with confidence.

Ultimately, a gallbladder-friendly lifestyle is not a restrictive set of rules but a holistic embrace of health-conscious choices. It is a narrative of renewal, resilience, and the power of understanding the gallbladder's role in the intricate dance of digestion.

As we bid farewell to the story of the Gallbladder Diet After Removal, let it serve as a reminder that the journey to recovery is unique for each individual. By making informed choices, fostering open communication with healthcare professionals, and approaching dietary adjustments with a positive mindset, one can embark on a path of healing, well-being, and a brighter, healthier future.

My Valued Reader,

I trust this culinary journey has not only ignited your passion for wholesome eating but has also become a haven of inspiration, solace, and invaluable insights. Each carefully curated recipe within this gallbladder diet after removal reflects a dedication to excellence, with a profound understanding of the comprehensive guide to the gallbladder diet

Crafted with meticulous attention to detail, these recipes go beyond the realm of mere sustenance; they are a testament to the art of nourishing the body and soul. Your reviews, experiences, and insights are treasures that guide me on this culinary odyssey.

Every evaluation is a stepping stone for refinement, as I aspire to tailor this food list to surpass your expectations. Let's engage in a dialogue that transcends the pages, creating a connection that resonates with your culinary preferences and well-being goals.

Warm Culinary Regards,

Tina Feldman